BEST NCLEX NOTES

DOCUMENTATION and LEADERSHIP

VOL.7

THE ART OF MASTERING NCLEX QUESTIONS

BY THE NCLEX MASTER

Best Nclex Notes

Psychosocial Strategies Vol.2

The Art of Mastering Nclex Questions

By the Nclex Master

Copyright© 2013 by Regional Hands Inc./ The Nclex Master

All rights reserved, including the right to reproduce this book or any portions in any form whatsoever, without permission in writing from the author.

Disclaimer: Due to the fact that the field of nursing is constantly changing, it is the reader and purchaser's responsibility for doing the research and studying on their own; also to obtain current healthcare information. Positive results are individualized. This book is in no way telling or recommending that it is not necessary to study course material provided by the school of their choosing in order to be a successful student and pass a test. This guide is solely for educational and entertainment purposes. Nor does the writer either or publisher of all volumes of this book assume any liability from injury, damage, negative test results, directly or indirectly to persons either or properties arising from the publication of this book.

Nor does the author wither or publisher have any financial gain from the publishers either or writers of recommended readings that are mentioned below.

My references and recommended reading material to utilize throughout nursing school: Saunders Comprehensive Review for the Nclex-RN examination by Linda Anne Silvestri edition 5. Philadelphia. 2005, WB Saunders. Saunders Strategies for Success for the Nclex-RN examination.

ISBN-13:9781494826635

ISBN-10:1494826631

In Loving Memory of Anderson F. Redding and Yvonne Lee

Volume Series:

Volume 1 Therapeutic Communication Strategies

Volume 2 Psychosocial Strategies

Volume 3 Physiological Strategies

Volume 4 Safe and Infection Strategies

Volume 5 Health Promotion Strategies

Volume 6 Pharmacology Strategies

Volume 7 Documentation and Leadership

CONTENTS

Introduction..9
Overview..11
Section 1 Report...12
Section 2 Calling the Doctor..16
Section 3 Documentation and Leadership Questions...............18
Section 4 Charting Pain..21
Section 5 Charting On A Patient On Hospice...................22
Section 6 Charting UTIs...23
Section 7 Charting Pneumonia.....................................24
Section 8 Charting COPD..25
Section 9 Charting CHF...26
Section 10 Charting On A Patient With Dyspnea..............27
Section11 Charting A Tracheostomy.............................28
Section 12 Charting A Patient With A GTUBE................29
Section 13 Charting Cast Care.....................................30
Section14 Charting A Bruise..31
Section 15 Charting Adverse Behaviors.........................32
Section 16 Charting On CVA..34
Section 17 Charting A Fracture....................................35
Section 18 Charting Neuro Checks...............................36
Section 19 Charting Antibiotics....................................37
Section 20 Charting Diarrhea......................................38

INTRODUCTION

Never before will you have access to helpful tips on Nclex, Hesi, and Ati questions the way I set forth. No matter what quarter you are attending in nursing school; you may have the same feelings that other students around you are experiencing. You also may be asking yourself…

"How well will I do on a nursing exam?"

"Why am I struggling when I am studying hard?"

"How can I master Nclex questions?"

"Will I pass Hesi and Ati exams?"

"Will I pass my school's exit exam?"

"Will I pass my state board exam on the first try?"

These are all valued questions and feelings to have. You can and will reach your goal of becoming a nurse. You just have to make sure you put the knowledge you gain each and every day to work in your best interest. Be positive; look in the mirror and say, "I am a nurse!"

I have experience some of the same feelings many of you have and I want you to know these 3 things:

I am You.

I was You.

I Am a Nurse.

This book is only one of many different guides that I will provide to you and other nursing students. In the near future there will be several more just like this, but with different topics and test taking strategies to look forward to.

The key is to master one guide at a time. This will help you to be more successful in answering not only nclex questions, but to know what the key elements you need to pay closer attention to, so you can be directed to the correct option.

Please do not take the information or recommendations I give you lightly. Make sure you study the material your professors give you and try your best to comprehend what you are reading. You may also find that you will have trouble understanding some content because it is hard to visualize something that you are not experienced in. When this happens, you really need to dig into nclex questions from the online material and the nclex books. When answering the questions, make sure you read the rationales to the questions. This is a great study tool and it provides you with follow up information that you may not have remembered or understood from your reading materials.

What you will find in all my guides are things you must know and also very helpful hints on the things you do not know to help you answer the questions. You have enough to read in the program itself, this is why my study guides are short and to the point, I am not here to teach you a nursing class, so please read every page carefully, so you can understand what I am referring to. Good Luck!

OVERVIEW

This guide is to help nursing students learn what pertinent information needs to be documented while giving care to their patient. Many new graduate nurses and current nurses may also benefit from this information. Although the healthcare systems are moving toward computerized charting to be utilizing in all healthcare settings, this documentation information is still needed for the nurse. You will still be held accountable for what you do and don't chart on. Make sure you always adhere to what the state board of nursing and your job's policies are for your scope of practice. Remember, if you didn't document; you didn't do it. You never know when you may be called in to court or sued.

As a nursing student and nurse you may have to care for a patient with issues that you are not familiar with or may have forgotten. This is where my document strategies for different diseases and disorders will help you to focus on the necessary content to help you document care.

In nursing school, the professors never gave us pertinent information to do focus charting on. When I got my first job, I was not given a list or information of different diseases or disorders on how to chart on them. I was doing paper charting and I found myself doing complete head to toe assessment charting on every patient I had to chart on for my shift. It should have been focus charting. We had to figure most of the information on our own or were notified by the supervisor about what needed to be focused on. If they would have provided a list, we could have had the opportunity to have the information on a clip board, so when we went to do our assessment we could have referred to the sheets of information to make sure certain information would not be left out.

With this issue at hand I have helped facilities and staff members implement charting procedures.

This is why I am giving you the ultimate start up documentation strategy guide to help you with things you need to pay close attention to. You can also expand your nursing notes beyond what I give you; each patient is a different patient and requires care that is suited for them.

Use this guide to help you in the areas of documentation that you need help with until you memorize what you need to do to be an effective caregiver.

How To Use This Guide:

Each Section will give you an overview of the things you need to look for in your patient and what you should focus your charting on.

For example if your patient has been diagnose with a urinary tract infection (UTI), you would go to the section UTI and read what things you should be looking for and what you should chart on.

You will be provided sections on what to ask the reporting off shift nurse and content before calling the doctor, along with helpful tips on when to choose document findings or notify doctor as your option to test questions.

Section 1
Report

I can't tell you how many times I've received report from a nurse and not get the necessary and correct information on a patient. We are only human and do make mistakes, but as nurses we are held accountable for errors that we may do. When I would travel to different facilities, most of the time the nurses were unable to tell me if a patient was on oxygen. If they did tell me the patient was receiving oxygen, I would ask how many liters and their response would be, "I'm not sure". Believe it or not, this happens quite often.

I know it is hard to believe that a nurse could oversee their patients all day and not know how many liters of oxygen their patient is receiving. There were also times when they would have the report sheet in their hand and just go down the list and say this patient was okay and no complaints. No other information about the patient would be given except, "He's okay; she's okay, and so on." How frustrating it would be at times, because as the nurse, if you strive to be the best nurse you can be, you will find yourself overworked because of the lack of communication and information given to you during change of shift report. In these types of situations you will find yourself going through your patient's chart to find out information that the off going shift nurse was unable to provide; making your shift start off in the wrong direction.

My goal is to help nursing students be aware that this does happen and not to let it get the best of you. I will give you a list of things that you should at least ask the off going shift nurse in report that I hope you will find helpful.

Things to ask during shift change:

- Patient's mental status
- Is patient cooperative with care?
- Last pain med, if given, what time?
- Where are usual complaints of pain located?
- Ask which patients receive their meds crushed
- Any patient NPO
- Is patient on oxygen and how many liters?
- Last biox reading
- Any respiratory issues?
- If acute setting ask why they are here, if long term care, you can refer to the chart if the nurse is unable to tell you.
- Are they diabetic?
- Last blood sugar
- Any patient with a foley
- Any patient with a tube feeding, the patient may have a g-tube or peg tube, but they take their meds orally, so ask. Don't assume.
- Any patient with an IV
- What is the feeding or IV solution used
- What is the flow rate on the pumps
- Any patient with wounds
- Any falls on shift, if so, who, what happen, are alarms in place, is patient on neuro checks, when is the next schedule assessment time? This is important to know because when report is over, you need to know if their next set of vital signs and neuro check needs to be implemented, so care is provided at the accurate times.
- Any labs that need to be done during shift or next shift

- Any labs that were drawn that needs to be looked for when they come back or reported to doctor if nurse was unable to notify doctor and family
- Any new doctor orders
- Any patient off unit and if so the estimated arrival time
- Any new admissions or discharges
- And any other issues or concerns the nurse had during their shift

This may seem like a lot, but really it isn't. In an acute setting you can refer to the updated kardex for information, but things do change and nurses do forget to tell you things in report. If you find yourself in this situation, you can either ask these questions from the beginning or wait until they are done if they did not provide you with basic report information. Things like how they toilet or transfer can also be given to you by a nurse's assistant working the floor in case you need to help someone to the bathroom. You are responsible for what goes on with your patients, so make sure you verify all information and not just take the word of the employees.

Section 2
Calling The Doctor

There is nothing worse than to be viewed as a nurse that doesn't know anything about the patient they are taking care of and a nurse who lacks organization skills when dealing with doctors.

Things to know and have before calling the doctor:

- Take patient's vital signs and assessment of the problem patient is experiencing.
- Have the patient MAR readily available in case doctor is giving you a medication order and ask you medication related questions about current meds the patient is currently receiving.
- If you are calling about abnormal labs, review the date of last labs obtained so you are able to tell the doctor what the abnormal lab is today and what it was on the most recent past lab date and what the doctor ordered the last time in case that information is pertinent for that particular doctor to know. Remember most doctors see hundreds of patient's and may not remember every single medication the patient had or currently is on. This will also alert you and the doctor if the labs are actually showing a mark improvement, a new issue that is going on, or if the patient's condition is getting worse.
- Know if the patient has any allergies on file and also ask the patient what they are allergic to. I'm telling you to check with the patient because I have an allergy and for some reason it was not in my chart and a nurse came to give me pain medication and when I asked her what it was I had to tell her I was allergic to it. Remember, sometimes things do fall through the cracks,

so always verify with the patient if they are able to tell you. Also, the doctor may give you a new order for an antibiotic that is contraindicated for the patient to receive. You are the eyes and ears for the doctor. The doctor may give an order but you are responsible once you give it. Remember, we are all a team and it takes a team to be an effective one. When it is all said and done, it is about the patient and not our egos. Don't get caught up into what someone else doesn't know, didn't tell you, or what they didn't do. We all make mistakes and if you were lucky enough to catch it, then it will benefit the patient in the long run.

- Remember when the doctor gives you an order, read the order back to him, ask for a start time/date and include the stop time/date, so other nurses will also know; especially for fluid restrictions and antibiotics. If the doctor or nurse practioner's new order is a steroid like prednisone, and you note there is not a tapered dose issued ask them about it. Get an accurate account how they want drug dosages to be implemented and chart it correctly. If a patient is a new admission ask for PRN pain med order. I can't tell you the countless times a patient had an elevated temp or mild pain and didn't have an order for Tylenol or there was no standing doctor order to give it.
- Also know the things I told you about regarding change of shift report in case you were given pertinent information that the doctor is not aware of.
- Know what it means when you see abnormal labs and what is usually done for a patient that has an abnormal lab and the signs and symptoms to watch out for. Don't be surprise if a doctor ask you what you think is going on.

I hope you find this information to be of some value to you. I know it will only make life a little less stressful for nursing students during the clinical rotations.

Section 3

Documentation and Leadership Questions

First step:
Know your normal lab ranges

Second step:
Know normal vital signs

Third step:
Know normal assessment findings

Fourth step:
Know the scope of practice for the unlicensed staff, LPN, and RN

These are important steps to know in order to answer questions that ask you who the RN will assign which client to.

HINT

Do not give LPNs unstable patients.
Do not give LPNs patients that need assessments done.
Do not give LPNs patients that are right out of surgery.
Do not give LPNs patients who need teaching done.

This information alone will help you to get numerous documentation questions right.

The RN will give the nursing assistant patients they can give a bed bath, shower, transfer in and out of a bed, chair, toilet, mouth care and feed unless the patient is having swallowing difficulty, vital signs unless there is a complication with that patient, emptying urine from a foley catheter, using a wheelchair to move a patient to another unit, and getting a patient dressed.

The RN will give the LPN/LVN patients that need a dressing change, medication by way of orally, rectally, or tube feeding, taking a patient blood sugar, giving IM or SubQ injections, suctioning, stable patients; this means no critically ill patients, and all the patients that a nursing assistant can take care of.

When to choose "Document Findings" as the option to a question:

- Any time the question you are reading gives you normal assessment findings and normal lab values
- When have a normal finding in a question and one of the options **DONOT** contain notify doctor, for example:

The question states: The nurse notice the laboratory report has come back with a potassium level 4.0 what will the nurse do next?

>Option 1. Document Findings
>Option 2. Call the family
>Option 3. Call the supervisor
>Option 4. Administer potassium IV

There are 3 clues in this question that you know to choose option1.

First Clue: Potassium level is normal

Second Clue: Option 1 and option 4 are opposites.

Third Clue: Option 2 and 3 are similar, so you know to eliminate those first.

Make sure you read the question and options thoroughly before choosing option.

HINT

If you are given an abnormal lab or an abnormal assessment that is critical in the question, and two of the four options to choose from is 1. Document findings or 2. Notify doctor, that is when you choose the option that contain notify doctor.

Majority of all questions you see that contain these two particular opposites, the correct option will be to notify the doctor.

Another helpful hint is if the question ask what the nurse would do immediately and you see notify doctor immediately, do not choose that as an answer. Read that again. Do you see the difference? Notifying the doctor and notifying the doctor immediately is two different things when the nurse is being asked what they should do immediately.

Find Nclex questions that contain these options and put this to the test and look up the correct option to put my strategy to test. You will find that this information is accurate.

Section 4
Charting Pain

Below are things you should be observing and include in your documentation:

- Location of pain
- Severity of pain on a scale 0-10, if they can't tell you what the pain level is but you notice facial grimacing, moaning, or groaning noted, document those findings.
- Type of pain patient is experiencing
- What makes pain worse
- What makes pain better
- Make sure you offer patient fluids, change of position, turn lights down or out, decrease noise or stimuli, offer back rub when appropriate, make sure patient is toileted and other protocol interventions your facility has in place before you give a pain medication.
- Document intervention
- Document pain medication used; make sure all medication is what is prescribed by the doctor.
- Document patient signs and symptoms after therapeutic time have lapsed. Chart the numerical value patient is able to state pain is after therapeutic techniques or administration of pain med. Chart if the patient is able to rest or sleep comfortably.

Make sure you let oncoming nurse know about patient's pain level, the location, and what medication was given and the time it was given.

Section 5
Charting On A Patient On Hospice

Below are things you should be observing and include in your documentation:

- The patient's level of consciousness (LOC)
- Lung sounds
- Respirations, rate and depth. This is important because it will alert you if the patient is experiencing any pain either or anxiety, or if the patient is about to be deceased.
- How the abdomen feels; is it firm soft, round, or distended?
- Bowel sounds
- Skin condition; is it warm, cool, pink, pale, cyanotic, any mottling, dry, moist/sweaty?
- Skin turgor
- Pain

Patient on hospice care are placed on comfort measures.
Drug of choice is Roxanol. Some doctors may order this to be given every two or four hours or the same prn. Be alert to patient LOC and respirations because this medication will suppress respirations although it relieves the anxiety and pain a patient may be experiencing.
Use your nursing judgment.

Section 6
Charting UTIs

Below are things you should be observing and include in your documentation:

- Urine Color; note if it is clear yellow, amber, or any sediment present.
- Amount of urine, if patient is voiding put a hat in the bathroom to collect urine. If patient has a foley catheter make sure staff is cleansing peri area properly. You may want to do a teaching session with staff to show them how to properly cleanse peri area with or without a foley present and how to use alcohol swab to cleanse drainage bag tube before and after urine is being drained and collected.
- Ask the patient if they are experiencing any burning, itching, or going to the bathroom frequently.
- Ask about pain or discomfort.
- Note if there is any increase in confusion.
- Take vital signs.
- Encourage fluids. Tell staff to offer patient fluids every two hours and you will offer the patient fluids on the hour that they are not doing it, that way the patient is drinking something every hour.
- Do I&O.
- Notify doctor of signs and symptoms of UTI
- Once you have an order for a lab to be drawn and once patient is on an antibiotic, make sure you do all the above and notify family of new orders. Note any allergies and make doctor aware. Obtain start time and date and stop time and date.
- Note any adverse reactions to antibiotic.

Section 7

Charting Pneumonia

Below are things you should be observing and include in your documentation:

- Vital signs
- Listen to lung sounds
- Check biox on the pulse oximetry
- Note an oxygen via nasal cannula and how many liters
- Note any Sweating
- Note any fever
- Note any chills
- Note any shortness of breath (SOB)
- Any cough
- Is the cough productive or nonproductive?
- Color of sputum
- Note antibiotic (ABT)
- Any adverse reactions to antibiotic
- Any pain
- Any difficulty breathing
- Respirations, are they even and unlabored?
- Elevate head of bed (HOB)
- Any confusion
- Any cyanosis

Make sure ABGs are within normal limits (WNL), the patient is able to cough and deep breath (C&DB), and patient is properly hydrated.

Section 8
Charting COPD

Below are things you should be observing and include in your documentation:

- Vital Signs
- Lung sounds
- Any SOB while at rest or change of position?
- Biox
- Any cough
- Is cough productive or nonproductive?
- Any sputum
- Note sputum's color; is it clear, thin, thick, yellow, green, or tan?
- Any wheezing heard
- Any confusion
- Any cyanosis
- Listen to apical pulse (AP), any irregularities heard?
- Any pain or discomfort?
- Elevate HOB

Most patients with COPD will be on nebulizer treatments and on low amount of oxygen via nasal cannula. These patients tend to like to sleep in a recliner.

Section 9
Charting CHF

Below are things you should be observing and include in your documentation:

- Vital signs especially blood pressure (BP)
- Apical pulse
- Any oxygen used
- Sweating
- Edema and it's location
- Is the edema pitting or nonpitting?
- If edema present note skin color, capillary refill, and mobility of the extremity that is affected and compare it to the unaffective side.
- Lung sounds
- Any SOB?
- Any dyspnea?
- Note peripheral pulses and if they are hard to palpate

Section 10

Charting on a patient with dyspnea

Below are things you should be observing and include in your documentation:

- Baseline vital signs and any changes
- Any cough present?
- Is it productive or nonproductive?
- Any sputum? The color of the sputum.
- Lung sounds
- Ask patient what they were doing when they began to have difficulty breathing.
- Was it sudden or gradual?
- Was it relieved while resting?
- LOC
- Restlessness
- Anxiety
- Fear
- Any cyanosis?
- Weakness
- Dizziness
- And notify doctor of findings

Make sure patient is stable before leaving patient to call doctor. Have call light in reach and if staff is available, have them sit with patient while you call doctor.

Section 11
Charting A Tracheostomy

Below are things you should be observing and include in your documentation:

- LOC
- Activity of patient
- Vital signs
- Method of communication
- Lung sounds
- Any difficulty breathing?
- Suctioning times and what secretions look like
- Note hypoxia
- Any cyanosis
- Biox
- I&O
- Note any bleeding around site and abnormal findings
- Dressing change, if already completed, change again when soiled and note findings
- Note any adverse emotions or behavior
- Any breathing treatments given and note respirations and lung sounds before and after treatment.
- Any anxiety?

When taking care of a person with a trach, make sure you use sterile technique with trach care and do not suction longer than 10 seconds.

Section 12

Charting A Patient With A GTube

Below are things you should be observing and include in your documentation:

- HOB at least 30 degrees
- Lung sounds
- Patency of tube
- Any residual noted?
- Skin around tube, any drainage, redness, or swelling noted?
- What does the abdomen feel like?
- Abdominal distention
- Bowel sounds
- Any diarrhea? If so, the doctor needs to be notified and the rate decreased. If giving a patient bolus feedings, you will need to slow the rate you are putting the feeding in by lowering the tube while putting nutritional supplement in tube
- Water flushes given per doctor order. Patients receiving feedings are at high risk for dehydration, so keeping up with the tube water flushes are very important part of care. Make sure water being used is not cold water.
- If patient has a dressing change to site, make sure it is dry and intact, and note any abnormal findings and notify doctor.
- Note if patient is tolerating the feeding well or not.

When taking care of a patient with a tube feeding, make sure the feeding is shut off 30 minutes prior to changing position of patient.

Section 13

Charting Cast Care

<u>Below are things you should be observing and include in your documentation:</u>
- Color of skin
- Temperature of skin, is area warm?
- Capillary refill
- Pulses bilaterally
- Any pain
- Any edema? If so, is it pitting or nonpitting? +1, +2, etc.
- Any tingling
- Numbness
- Notify doctor of abnormal findings

Section 14
Charting A Bruise

Below are things you should be observing and include in your documentation:

- The location of the bruise
- The color
- Measure bruise and note the size, follow your job's policy and procedure regarding when to notify supervisor for bruise sizes and state reportable sizes.
- Pain
- Tenderness
- Any swelling
- Ask patient if they remembered what happen and also ask workers that were taking care of patient if they know what happen.
- Note any interventions that took place, for example any ice or elevation of extremity noted.
- Any change in behavior
- Make sure patient didn't fall, if so start neuro check if unwitnessed and incident report. Follow your job's policy regarding falls and incident reporting.
- Check patient's MAR to see if bruise could be related to patient taking Coumadin; doctor needs to be notified.
- Notify family

Section 15

Charting Adverse Behaviors

Below are things you should be observing and include in your documentation:

- Describe the situation
- Describe the location
- People involved
- The time it took place
- Anxious behavior
- Negative statements
- Repetitive statements
- Repetitive questions
- Repetitive health complaints
- Verbal abuse
- Physical aggression, hitting, slapping, or kicking
- Any exposure of body parts
- Agitation
- Anxiety
- Sadness
- Crying; tearfulness
- Foul language
- Spitting at others
- Lack of interest during activities
- Lack of involvement in care
- Social isolation
- Any safety concerns

- What interventions were implemented
- Behavior forms initiated or filled out if patient already has one that exist.

Make sure social services form is filled out, doctor is notified, any new orders are completed, family is notified, and provide one on one if necessary.

Section 16
Charting On CVA

Below are things you should be observing and include in your documentation:

- Vital signs
- LOC
- Airway patency
- Speech, is it slurred?
- Facial features
- Asymmetrical face
- Memory
- Crying
- Lung sounds
- Coughing
- Swallowing difficulty
- Inability to perform ADLs
- Assistive devices
- Crush meds
- Puree diet or mechanical soft
- Thicken liquids; nectar thick
- Speech therapy

Section 17
Charting A Fracture

Below are things you should be observing and include in your documentation:

- Joint flexibility
- Muscle strength
- Range of motion (ROM)
- Assistive devices
- Pain
- Capillary refill
- Pulses
- Tingling
- Numbness
- Edema
- Compare extremities
- Appropriate alignment

Section 18

Charting Neuro Checks

Below are things you should be observing and include in your documentation:

- Any numbness
- Any tingling
- Any cold sensations
- Any hot sensations
- Any tremors
- Pupil size
- LOC
- Appearance of toes
- Appearance of fingers
- Appearance of hands
- Appearance of feet
- Any complaints patient may be experiencing
- Notify doctor
- Notify family

Section 19

Charting Antibiotics

Below are things you should be observing and include in your documentation:

- Vital signs; especially watch the temperature
- The reason patient is receiving the ABT
- Make sure culture and sensitivity is obtain prior to receiving ABT if possible
- Reassess patient to see if symptoms are getting better
- Any adverse reactions to meds
- Hives
- Rash
- Itching
- Swelling
- Redness
- Flushing
- Encourage fluids

Section 20
Charting Diarrhea

Below are things you should be observing and include in your documentation:

- How many loose stools
- The color
- Put a hat in the toilet and measure the amount
- Note any signs and symptoms of dehydration; dry mucous membranes, etc.
- Skin turgor
- Bowel sounds
- Abdominal distention
- Any pain
- Any tenderness
- The cause
- Notify the doctor
- Initiate a C-Diff culture per job's policy and procedure and doctor order
- Place patient on contact isolation as a preventive measure before test results come back
- Possible private room if one available
- Stress handwashing techniques with all staff members
- Put soiled linen in proper disposal containers

If you have gotten this volume in paperback you may also want to get it on your kindle or download it to your ipad or iphone. This way you will be able to use this guide at clinical or work when you take care of a patient with any of these signs or symptoms.

Always know what normal finding is so you know when something abnormal is occurring and what the patient baseline vitals are.

www.ingramcontent.com/pod-product-compliance
Lightning Source LLC
Chambersburg PA
CBHW070725180526
45167CB00004B/1621